The Optimum

Dr Sebi Cancer Diet:

Discover how to cure cancer naturally with the Dr Sebi Alkaline Diet Method

(Nutritional and Medical Guide)

COPYRIGHT PAGE

Table of Contents

Introduction

What all types of cancer have in common is that the cancer cells are abnormal and multiply out of control. However, there are often great differences between different types of cancer.

Some grow and spread more quickly than others and some are easier to treat than others, particularly if diagnosed at an early stage.

Some respond much better than others to chemotherapy, radiotherapy, or other treatments, while some have a better outlook (prognosis) than others. For some types of cancer there is a very good chance of being cured. For some types of cancer, the outlook is poor.

So, cancer is not just one condition. In each case it is important to know exactly what type of cancer has developed, how large it has become, whether it has spread and how well the particular type of cancer responds to various treatments. This will enable you to get reliable information on treatment options and outlook.

What is cancer?

Cancer is a large group of diseases that occur when abnormal cells divide rapidly and can spread to other tissue and organs.

These rapidly growing cells may cause tumors. They may also disrupt the body's regular function.

Cancer is one of the leading causes of death in the world. According to the World Health Organization (WHO), cancer accounted for almost 1 in 6 deaths in 2020. Experts are working hard to test out new cancer treatments every day.

Types of Cancer and How They Differ

The are more than 200 different types of cancer, each of which is grouped under a larger cancer category like carcinomas, myelomas, leukemias, and so forth. Because of this, simply learning that you or someone you know has cancer doesn't tell you a whole lot. Cancer is not a single disease, and different types of cancers have different origins, treatments, and prognoses.

Some cancers are grouped based on the cell, tissue, or body region where they start. Others types of cancer are described by their genetic profile, tumor grade, or cancer stage. Learn all about them here.

Primary vs. Metastatic

Primary cancer refers to the original tumor in the body. In some cases, cancer may start and be treated effectively enough to stay in the area in which it began.

That definition is pretty straightforward. Confusion over the term tends to lie in its use for cancer that has spread to another part of the body.

When a cancer travels (metastasizes) from its original site, it is named for the type of cancer cell or organ in which it began not for the region of the body it has spread to. For example, if breast cancer begins in the breast and later spreads to the lung, it would not be called lung cancer. Instead, it would be referred to as primary breast cancer metastatic to the lungs.

A diagnosis of "invasive" cancer does not mean that your cancer has spread. Even a stage 1 cancer is referred to in this way, based on the appearance of the tumor under a microscope.

You may also hear the term secondary cancer. This is a second primary cancer unrelated to the original tumor that is found in another part of the body. In other words, the additional cancer just so happens to have occurred at the same time as the first cancer, but it did not happen because of spreading of cancer cells.

Healthcare providers are unable to determine where a cancer began in about 3% to 5% of cases, and only find evidence of cancer where it has spread. This is referred to as an unknown primary, or cancer of unknown origin, with metastasis to the location where the cancer is discovered.

Primary vs. Secondary Cancers

By Cell or Tissue Type

The name for many cancers derives from the type of cells in which the cancer begins. For example, you may have been told you have kidney cancer, but kidney cancers can differ significantly based on the type of kidney cell in which a tumor starts.

There are six major types of cancer based on cell type:

- Carcinomas
- Sarcomas
- Myelomas
- Leukemias
- Lymphomas
- Mixed types (including blastomas)

Carcinomas

Carcinomas are the most common cell type of cancer, accounting for 80% to 90% of cancers. These cancers arise in epithelial cells, which include the cells of the skin and those that line body cavities and cover organs.

Carcinomas may be further broken down into:

- Adenocarcinomas: Adenocarcinomas begin in glandular cells that manufacture fluids, such as breast milk.
- Squamous cell carcinomas: Examples of squamous cells include those in the top layer of the skin, the upper portion of the esophagus and airways, and the lower portion of the cervix and vagina.

- Basal cell carcinomas: Basal cells are only present in the skin and are the deepest layer of skin cells.

- Transitional cell carcinomas: Transitional cells are epithelial cells that are "stretchy" and are present in the bladder and parts of the kidney.

In addition to these more specific cell types, carcinomas may be named based on their location. For example, breast carcinomas that arise in the milk ducts would be referred to as ductal carcinomas, whereas those that arise in the lobules are considered lobular carcinomas.

Carcinomas are the only cancer cell type that have a noninvasive phase, and therefore are the only cancers for which screening is routinely done.

Cancers that are still "contained" and have not spread through the basement membrane are referred to as carcinoma in situ (CIN). Cancer detected at this early, pre-invasive stage has an excellent prognosis.

Sarcomas

Sarcomas are cancers of the bone and soft tissues of the body that are made up of cells called mesenchymal cells. This type of cancer affects bone, muscles (both skeletal and smooth muscle), tendons, ligaments, cartilage, blood vessels, nerves, synovial tissues (joint tissues), and fatty tissues.

Examples of sarcomas include:

- Osteosarcoma (bone cancers)
- Chondrosarcoma (cartilage cancers)

- Liposarcoma (fatty tissue cancers)
- Rhabdomyosarcoma (skeletal muscle cancers)
- Leiomyosarcoma (smooth muscle cancers)
- Angiosarcoma (blood vessel cancers)
- Mesothelioma (cancers of the mesothelium, the tissues that line the chest and abdominal cavities)
- Fibrosarcoma (cancers of fibrous tissues)
- Glioma and astrocytoma (cells of the connective tissue in the brain)

What's In a Name?

Generally speaking, cancerous tumors usually include the name of the particular cell type in which they began followed by "sarcoma." For example, a benign bone tumor might be called an osteoma, but a malignant tumor, an osteosarcoma.

Myelomas

Myeloma, also called multiple myeloma, is a cancer of cells in the immune system known as plasma cells. Plasma cells are the cells that manufacture antibodies.

Leukemias

Leukemias are cancers of the blood cells, and they originate in the bone marrow. Among blood-related cancers, leukemias are considered "liquid cancers" in contrast to myelomas and lymphomas. Since these cancers involve cells that circulate in the bloodstream, they are often treated like solid cancers that have spread. Examples include:

- Lymphocytic leukemias: These are cancers of white blood cells known as lymphocytes.

- Myelocytic leukemias: These are cancers of mature or immature cells known as myelocytes, such as neutrophils.

Both lymphocytic and myelocytic leukemias have forms that progress quickly (acute) and forms that take longer to develop (chronic).

Lymphomas

Lymphomas are a type of cancer that arises from cells of the immune system. These cancers may arise in lymph nodes or from extranodal sites such as the spleen, stomach, or testicles. These are broken down into:

- Hodgkin lymphoma
- Non-Hodgkin lymphoma

Blood-Related vs. Solid Cancer Types

Cancers may also be referred to as "solid" or blood-related cancers. Blood-related cancers include leukemias, lymphomas, and myelomas, while solid cancers include all others.

Mixed Types

It's not uncommon for a cancer to have characteristics of more than one type of tissue. Cancer cells differ from normal cells in many ways, one of which is referred to as differentiation.

Some cancers can look very much like the normal cells in which they originate. They are called well-differentiated tumors. Others may bear little resemblance to normal cells. You may see them described as undifferentiated on a pathology report.

In addition to this, most tumors are heterogeneous. This means that the cells in one part of a tumor may look very different from cells in another part of a tumor.

For example, a lung cancer may have some cells that look like adenocarcinoma and others that appear to be squamous cell carcinoma. On a pathology report, this is called adenosquamous features.

Blastomas are a type that is sometimes separated out from the rest. These are cancers that occur in embryonic cells cells that have not yet chosen a path to become epithelial cells or mesenchymal cells.

By Body Part/System

Types of cancer are also often described by the organs or organ systems in which they begin.

Central Nervous System Cancers

Central nervous system cancers include those that originate in tissues of either the brain or the spinal cord. Cancers that spread to the brain are not considered brain cancers, but rather brain metastases, and are far more common than primary brain cancers.

Cancers that commonly spread to the brain include:

- Lung cancer
- Breast cancer
- Melanoma

Unlike tumors in other regions of the body, brain cancers do not often spread outside of the brain. Overall, however, the incidence of brain cancer has been increasing in recent years. Improving overall cancer survival rates means more metastatic cases (the longer someone lives with cancer, the greater the chances of it spreading).

Gliomas and Brain Cancer

Head and Neck Cancers

Head and neck cancers can affect any region of the head and neck, from the tongue to the vocal cords. In the past, these cancers were most commonly seen in people who were both heavy drinkers and smokers.

In recent years, however, human papillomavirus (HPV) has become an important cause of these cancers, with close to 10,000 people developing HPV-related head and neck cancers each year in the United States alone.

Two such cancers are:

- Oral cancer: Roughly 60-70% of all head and neck cancers are oral cancers. These cancers may involve the mouth, tongue, tonsils, throat (pharynx), and the nasal passageways.
- Laryngeal cancer (cancer of the vocal cords)

Breast Cancers

Many people are aware that breast cancer is an all-too-common cancer in women, but it's important to point out that men get breast cancer also.

Approximately 1 in 100 breast cancers occur in men. The most common type of breast cancer is ductal carcinoma.

Since most breast cancers are carcinomas, they may sometimes be detected before they have become invasive. This is considered carcinoma in situ, or stage 0 breast cancer.

Breast cancer stages 1 through 4 are invasive stages of the disease. You may hear these more specific names:

- Ductal carcinoma in situ of the breast (DCIS) and lobular carcinoma in situ (LCIS): Carcinoma in situ is the earliest stage at which breast cancer can be detected and is considered stage 0. These cancers have not yet penetrated through the basement membrane and are considered non-invasive. They are most often detected when a biopsy is done for an abnormality on a screening mammogram.

- Invasive (infiltrating) breast cancer (both ductal and lobular): Once a breast cancer penetrates through the basement membrane, it is considered invasive.

- Inflammatory breast cancer: Inflammatory breast cancer, in contrast to other breast cancers, does not usually present as a lump. Rather, the early stages of the disease look like a redness and rash on the breast.

- Male breast cancer: When breast cancer occurs in men, it is more likely that there is a genetic component. A family history of breast cancer should prompt a discussion with your healthcare provider.

Respiratory Cancers

Cancers of the lung and bronchial tubes are the leading cause of cancer deaths in both men and women in the United States. While smoking is a risk factor for these diseases, lung cancer occurs in never-smokers as well. In fact, lung cancer in these individuals is the sixth-leading cause of cancer deaths in the United States.

Lung cancer rates are decreasing overall, likely related to a decrease in smoking. But they are increasing in young adults, especially young, never-smoking women. The reason is not understood and remains under study at this time.

Types you may hear about include:

- Non-small cell lung cancer: Subtypes of non-small cell lung cancer (responsible for around 80-85% of lung cancers) include lung adenocarcinoma, squamous cell carcinoma of the lungs, and large cell lung cancer.
- Small cell lung cancer: Small cell lung cancer accounts for around 15% of lung cancers and is more likely to occur in people who have smoked.
- Mesothelioma: Mesothelioma is a cancer of the pleural mesothelium, the lining surrounding the lungs. It is strongly linked with exposure to asbestos.

Digestive System Cancers

Digestive tract cancers may occur anywhere from the mouth to the anus. Most of these cancers are adenocarcinomas, with squamous cell carcinomas occurring in the upper esophagus and most distant portion of the anus. Types include:

- Esophageal cancer: The most common form of esophageal cancer has changed in recent years. Whereas squamous cell esophageal cancer (often related to smoking and drinking) was once the most common form of the disease, it has been surpassed by esophageal adenocarcinoma (often related to long-standing acid reflux).
- Stomach cancer: Stomach cancer is uncommon in the United States, but is a common type of cancer worldwide.

- Pancreatic cancer: Pancreatic cancer is less common than some other cancers, but is the fourth most common cause of cancer-related deaths in both men and women. It is most often diagnosed in the later stages of the disease, when surgery is unfortunately no longer possible.

- Liver cancer: Cancer metastatic to the liver is much more common than primary liver cancer. Risk factors for liver cancer include alcohol abuse and chronic infections with hepatitis B or C.

- Colon cancer: Colon cancer is often referred to as colorectal cancer and includes both cancers of the rectum and the upper colon. It is the third leading cause of cancer deaths in both men and women.

- Anal cancer: Anal cancer differs from colon cancer both in treatments and causes.

Studies now show that 91% of all anal cancers are associated with HPV virus, the majority linked to just two subtypes (HPV-16 and HPV-18).

Causes and Risk Factors of HPV

Urinary System Cancers

The genitourinary system involves the kidneys, the bladder, the tubes connecting the kidneys and bladder (called the ureters), and the urethra (the passageway out from the bladder). This system also includes structures such as the prostate gland. Types include:

- Kidney cancer: The most common types of kidney cancer include renal cell carcinoma (around 90% of cases), transitional cell carcinoma, and Wilms' tumor in children.

- Bladder cancer: Roughly half of bladder cancers are caused by tobacco exposure. Those who work with dyes and paints are also at higher risk.
- Prostate cancer: Prostate is the second leading cause of cancer death in men, but now has a very high five-year survival rate.

Reproductive System Cancers

Reproductive organ cancers may occur in men and women. Ovarian cancer is the fifth most common cause of cancer deaths in women, and though curable in the early stages, is often diagnosed when it has already spread. Types include:

- Testicular cancer

- Ovarian cancer (including germ cell tumors)
- Uterine cancer (also called endometrial cancer)
- Fallopian tube cancer
- Cervical cancer

Endocrine Cancers

The endocrine system is a series of glands that produce hormones and, as such, may have symptoms of an over- or underproduction of these hormones.

Most endocrine cancers, with the exception of thyroid cancer, are fairly rare. A combination of different endocrine cancers may run in families and is referred to as multiple endocrine neoplasia, or MEN.

The incidence of thyroid cancer is increasing in the United States at a higher rate, but the survival rate for many of these cancers also is high.

Bone and Soft Tissue Cancers

In contrast to primary bone and soft tissue cancers, which are uncommon, cancer that is metastatic to bone is common. Bone cancer, either primary or metastatic, often presents with symptoms of pain or of a pathologic fracture a fracture that occurs in a bone that is weakened by the presence of tumor. Types include:

- Osteosarcoma
- Kaposi's sarcoma: Kaposi's sarcoma is a soft tissue cancer often seen in people with HIV/AIDS.
- Ewing's sarcoma: Ewing's sarcoma is a bone cancer that primarily affects children.

Blood-Related Cancers

Blood-related cancers include both those involving blood cells and those involving solid tissue of the immune system, such as lymph nodes.

The risk factors for blood-related cancers differ somewhat from solid cancers in that environmental exposures as well viruses, such as the Epstein-Barr virus, play a significant role.

Blood-related cancers are the most common cancers in children. They include:

- Hodgkin lymphoma
- Non-Hodgkin lymphoma
- Acute lymphocytic leukemia
- Chronic lymphocytic leukemia
- Acute myelogenous leukemia

- Chronic myelogenous leukemia
- Myeloma

Skin Cancers

Skin cancers are often separated into two primary groups: melanoma and non-melanoma. While non-melanoma skin cancers are much more common, melanomas are responsible for most skin cancer deaths.

Examples of skin cancers include:

- Basal cell carcinoma
- Squamous cell carcinoma of the skin
- Skin cancer is the most common type of cancer overall in the United States, according to the Centers for Disease Control and Prevention (CDC).

Other Classification Methods

In addition to grouping cancers in the above ways, tumors are often classified by:

- Tumor grade: Grade is a measure of the aggressiveness of a tumor. A grade 1 tumor is less aggressive, and the cells may closely resemble the normal cells in which the cancer began. A grade 3 tumor, in contrast, is usually more aggressive, and the cells look very different than normal cells.

- Tumor stage: Tumors are staged in different ways, but many are given a number between 1 and 4, with 4 being the most advanced stage of the cancer.

- Non-hereditary cancer vs. hereditary cancer: Some cancers are referred to as hereditary cancers. For example, around 5-10% of breast cancers are referred to as such. There is much overlap, and genetics play a role in many cancers.

- DNA/molecular profiles: As our understanding of genetics improves, tumors are more frequently being classified in terms of genetic profile. For example, some lung cancers have EGFR mutations, while others have ALK rearrangements.

Signs and Symptoms of Cancer

Reviewing cancer symptoms can be surprising and worrying. While there are several common symptoms of cancer, there are few that are specific to this group of diseases. Aside from those you may immediately associate with cancer (e.g., a breast lump or skin changes), symptoms such as bloating, persistent cough, and others can also occur. Of course, these vague symptoms may also indicate something else entirely.

Symptoms of cancer vary widely depending on the type of disease. For instance, a tumor can invade nearby structures and affect their function, or press on nerves (e.g., ovarian cancer may cause constipation by pressing on the colon; lung cancer may cause hoarseness by pressing on a nerve as it travels through the chest). In addition, cancer often causes metabolic changes that result in generalized symptoms such as fatigue, weight loss, and an overall sense of being unwell.

Recognizing the early symptoms of cancer can help you have the best chance for early detection and effective treatment.

Frequent Symptoms

While it's important to remember that each of the most common symptoms of cancer can have other causes, it's best to talk to your healthcare provider about any that you experience.

These are the 14 most common symptoms of cancer:

- Unintentional or unexplained weight loss
- Lumps, bumps, or enlarged lymph nodes
- Night sweats
- Abnormal vaginal bleeding
- Changes in your bowel movements
- Blood in your stool or rectal bleeding
- Persistent cough
- Shortness of breath
- Pain occurring anywhere in your body, especially a pain felt as a deep ache

- Persistent, severe fatigue
- Skin changes
- Abdominal swelling or bloating
- Blood in your urine
- Difficulty swallowing

Your gut feeling can be an important "early symptom" of cancer. Upon learning of their diagnosis of cancer, many people state that they knew something was wrong. A large 2016 study confirmed this finding, at least with colorectal cancer. The third most commonly reported symptom prior to diagnosis was "feeling different."

Some of these symptoms are specific to certain types of cancer, while others may occur in several types.

Unexplained Weight Loss

Unintentional weight loss is defined as the loss of 5% of body weight over a six- to 12-month period without trying. This is equivalent to a 130-pound woman losing 6 or 7 pounds, or a 200-pound man losing roughly 10 pounds of weight. Though many people may welcome dropping a few pounds, it's important to see your healthcare provider if you do unexpectedly lose weight.

Cancer is the cause of unintentional weight loss at least 25% of the time. While weight loss is more likely to occur in advanced cancers, it can occur in early-stage cancers as well.

Cancer can cause weight loss in several ways:

- Changes in the metabolic activity of the body caused by cancer may increase daily calorie needs.
- Cancers such as colon cancer can cause people to become full faster when eating, reducing their overall consumption.
- Other cancers may interfere with eating by causing nausea or difficulty swallowing.
- Sometimes people with cancer may simply not feel well enough to eat as they normally would.
- The syndrome of cancer cachexia, which includes weight loss as well as muscle wasting, is not only a symptom of cancer but is considered the direct cause of death in up to 20% of people with cancer.

Why Unexplained Weight Loss Is Concerning

Lumps and Bumps

A lump or thickening anywhere on your body that does not have an explanation is an important first symptom of cancer.

Breast lumps could be cancer but could also easily be benign breast cysts or fibroadenomas. There are less common signs of breast cancer as well, and symptoms such as redness, thickening, or an orange-peel appearance to the breast should be addressed.

It's important to see your healthcare provider if you have any changes in your breast tissue, even if you've had a normal mammogram. Mammograms miss around 20% of breast cancers.

Testicular lumps may be a symptom of testicular cancer, and just as women are encouraged to do monthly self-breast exams, men are encouraged to do monthly testicular self-exams.

Enlarged lymph nodes may be the first sign of cancer especially lymphomas and can occur in many regions of the body. In fact, enlarged lymph nodes are one of the key warning signs of lymphoma.

Enlarged lymph nodes may be a sign of many solid tumors as well. Lymph nodes function as "dumpsters" in some ways. The first cancer cells to escape a tumor tend to be caught in the lymph nodes closest to a tumor, and many cancers spread to nearby lymph nodes before spreading further in the body.

Other bumps, thickenings, or even bruises out of proportion to an injury should be evaluated by your healthcare provider.

Night Sweats

Night sweats are a common symptom of cancer, especially leukemias and lymphomas. Night sweats that occur with cancer are not simply "hot flashes." They are often drenching to the point that people need to get out of bed and change their pajamas, sometimes repeatedly. Unlike hot flashes, which may occur at any time of the day or night, night sweats are more common when sleeping.

Night sweats in men should always be evaluated by a healthcare provider. While this can be an important symptom of cancer in women as well, it can be hard to differentiate what is "normal" or not in women, especially those who are in the early stages of menopause.

Night Sweats and Cancer

Abnormal Vaginal Bleeding

Abnormal vaginal bleeding can be a sign of cancer but certainly has many benign causes as well. Abnormal bleeding can take many forms, including:

- Bleeding between periods
- Periods that are heavier or lighter than usual
- Bleeding after sex
- Bleeding after you have completed menopause

Cancers of the uterus, cervix, and vagina may cause bleeding directly related to a tumor. Hormonal changes due to cancers, such as ovarian cancer, may also cause changes in your menstrual cycle.

Every woman is different, and the most important symptoms are those that represent a change in what is normal for you.

Changes in Bowel Habits

If you experience changes in your bowel movements, whether in color, consistency, or frequency, talk to your healthcare provider. Symptoms of colon cancer can range from diarrhea to constipation, but what is most concerning is something that is out of the norm for you.

Rectal Bleeding

If you see blood in your stool you will likely be worried, but as with other possible cancer symptoms, there are many benign causes as well.

The color of the blood is sometimes useful in determining the origin of the blood (but not the cause). Bleeding from the lower colon (left colon) and rectum is often bright red. That from the upper colon (right colon) and small intestine is often dark red, brown, or black. And blood from higher up, for example, the esophagus or stomach, is very dark and often resembles coffee grounds.

Other causes of rectal bleeding include hemorrhoids, anal fissures, and colitis, but an important point to note is that even if you have these other conditions it does not mean that you don't also have colon cancer. In fact, some types of colitis are a risk factor for colon cancer.9

If you have this symptom, make sure to see your healthcare provider even if you think there is a reasonable cause.

Persistent Cough

A persistent cough may be a symptom of lung cancer; roughly half of people with the disease have a chronic cough at the time of diagnosis. It could also be a sign of a cancer that has spread to the lungs, such as breast cancer, colon cancer, kidney cancer, or prostate cancer.

A cough can be caused by a narrowing of the airways caused by a tumor, or as the result of infections that arise as a result of tumors in the lungs. Of course, respiratory conditions such as chronic obstructive pulmonary disease (COPD) must also be considered.

Shortness of Breath

Shortness of breath is one of the leading early symptoms of lung cancer. While you may associate lung cancer with a chronic cough, the most common symptoms of lung cancer have changed over time.

A few decades ago the most common types of the disease tended to grow near the large airways in the lungs; a location that frequently caused a cough and coughing up blood. Today, the most common form of lung cancer lung adenocarcinoma tends to grow in the outer regions of the lungs. These tumors can grow quite large before they are detected, and often cause shortness of breath with activity as their first symptom.

Other Possible Causes of Shortness of Breath

Chest, Abdominal, Pelvic, Back, or Head Pain
Pain occurring anywhere in your body could be a possible symptom of cancer. If you have any unexplained pain that persists, especially pain you would describe as a deep ache, talk to your healthcare provider.

Head Pain

Headaches are the most common symptom of brain cancer or tumors that have spread (metastasized) to the brain, but certainly most headaches are not due to cancer.

The classic headache due to a brain tumor is severe, at its worst in the morning, and progresses over time. These headaches may worsen with activities such as coughing or bearing down for a bowel movement, and may occur on one side only. People with a headache related to a brain tumor frequently have other symptoms, such as nausea and vomiting, weakness of one side of the body, or new-onset seizures. However, brain tumors can also cause headaches that are indistinguishable from a tension headache, and may be the only sign that a tumor is present.

Cancer spread to the brain (brain metastases) are seven times more common than primary brain tumors and cause similar symptoms. Cancers most likely to spread to the brain include breast cancer, lung cancer, bladder cancer, and melanoma. It's not uncommon for people with brain metastases, especially those with small cell lung cancer, to have symptoms related to a tumor in the brain before they have symptoms due to the primary cancer.

Back Pain

The most common cause of back pain is a back strain, but back pain that persists and doesn't have an obvious cause could be a symptom of cancer as well. Back pain related to cancer is often (but not always) worse at night, does not improve when you lie down, and may worsen with a deep breath or during bowel movements.

Back pain can be caused by tumors in the chest, abdomen, or pelvis, or by metastases to the spine from other cancers.

Shoulder Pain

Pain that is felt in the shoulders or shoulder blades can easily be due to a muscle strain, but it can also be an important early symptom of cancer. Referred pain from lung cancer, breast cancer, and lymphomas, as well as metastases from other cancers, may cause aching in the shoulders or shoulder blade pain.

Chest Pain

There are many causes of chest pain, with heart disease often being a prime suspect. Unexplained chest pain can be a symptom of cancer as well. Though the lung does not have nerve endings, pain that feels like "lung pain" is present in a large number of people who are diagnosed with lung cancer.

Abdominal or Pelvic Pain

As with pain in other regions of the body, abdominal pain and pelvic pain are most often associated with conditions other than cancer. One of the difficulties with pain in the abdomen and pelvis, however, is that it's often hard to determine where the pain begins.

When to See a Healthcare Provider for Abdominal Pain

Fatigue

Unlike ordinary tiredness, cancer fatigue is often much more persistent and disabling. Some people describe this tiredness as "total body tiredness" or exhaustion. It's not something you can push through with a good night of rest or a strong cup of coffee. The hallmark of this kind of fatigue is that it significantly interferes with your life.

There are many ways in which cancer can cause fatigue. The growth of a tumor, in general, can be taxing for your body. Other symptoms of cancer such as shortness of breath, anemia, pain, or a decreased level of oxygen in your blood (hypoxia) can cause fatigue as well.

If you find that fatigue is disrupting your normal activities, make sure to talk to your healthcare provider.

Skin Changes

There are many types of "skin changes" that could be a symptom of skin cancer. Some of these include new spots on your skin (no matter the color), a sore that does not heal, or a change in a mole or freckle.

While skin cancers such as basal cell carcinoma and squamous cell carcinoma are more common, melanoma is responsible for the majority of deaths from skin cancer.

Familiarize yourself with the ABCDEs of melanoma, which cover aspects of skin changes (asymmetry, borders, diameter, and more) that may indicate skin cancer. Though a less-than-clinical distinction, many experts note that even something you consider "funny looking" could be a sign of skin cancer.

It's worth noting that melanomas are often first noticed by someone else. If your loved one has a suspicious looking skin spot, don't be afraid to say something.

ABCDEs of Melanoma

Bloating (Abdominal Distension)

Abdominal swelling or bloating may be a first symptom of several cancers, including ovarian cancer, pancreatic cancer, and colon cancer.

You may feel a fullness in your abdomen, or may note that your clothes are tighter around the middle even though you haven't gained weight.

Ovarian cancer has been coined the "silent killer" as symptoms often occur late in the disease, and then are frequently dismissed as due to something else.

It's been found that bloating is a common symptom of ovarian cancer, but women often attribute this symptom to weight gain or other causes. Likewise, constipation, pain with intercourse, constipation, and frequent urination can be symptoms of ovarian cancer, but are often first attributed to other causes.

If you notice any of these symptoms, talk to your healthcare provider. Ovarian cancer can be treatable when caught early.

Blood in Urine

Blood in your urine can be a symptom of bladder cancer. Even a slight pink tinge to your urine warrants a visit to your healthcare provider. This is extra important if you have a history of smoking, as the habit is responsible for at least half of bladder cancer cases.

Difficulty Swallowing

Difficulty swallowing, also known as dysphagia, can be a symptom of cancer. It is often the first symptom of esophageal cancer due to narrowing of the esophagus.

Since the esophagus travels through the area between the lungs (called the mediastinum), tumors in this region such as lung cancer and lymphomas often cause this symptom as well.

Why Swallowing Difficulties Can Occur

Rare Symptoms

There are several less common, but no less important symptoms that may alert you to the presence of a cancer. Some of these include:

- Blood clots: There are many risk factors for blood clots in the legs known as deep vein thrombosis (DVT). In recent years, it's been noted that one of these factors can be a previously undiagnosed cancer. It is important to know the symptoms of DVTs not just because of this, however, but because they often break off and travel to the lungs, something known as a pulmonary embolus.

- Urinary changes: Changes in urination such as frequency or difficulty starting your stream can be an early symptom of cancer.

- Heartburn or indigestion: Chronic heartburn due to gastroesophageal reflux disease (GERD) is an important cause of esophageal cancer. If you have long-standing heartburn, talk to your healthcare provider about screening.

- Shingles: Shingles, a condition caused by reactivation of the chickenpox virus, can be a symptom of underlying cancer.

- Depression: New-onset depression is a fairly common early symptom of cancer.

- Fractures with minimal trauma: When cancers spread to bones they can weaken them so that fractures occur with minimal trauma. A fracture that occurs in a bone weakened by cancer is called a pathologic fracture.

- Easy bruising: Cancers that infiltrate the bone marrow can reduce the number of platelets in your blood. Decreased platelets, in turn, can result in easy bruising.

- White patches in your mouth: White patches on the gums or tongue (called leukoplakia) could be an early symptom of oral cancers, and many healthcare providers now routinely screen for this during regular dental exams. Whereas smoking and drinking were the prime culprits causing these cancers in the past, many are now believed to be caused by infections with the human papillomavirus (HPV).

- Finally, some cancers cause unique symptoms based on compounds they produce and secrete. These symptoms referred to as paraneoplastic syndromes may present with symptoms caused by the actions of those compounds.

For example, some lung cancers produce a hormone-like substance that raises the calcium level in the blood. Symptoms of hypercalcemia (high blood calcium), such as muscle aches, may, therefore, be the first symptom of cancer.

Sub-Groups and Complications

It's important not to dismiss symptoms due to a lack of risk factors. For example, breast cancer does occur in men, as well as many women without a family history of the disease. Lung cancer does occur in people who have never smoked. And colon cancer does occur in young men and women.

If you have any symptoms, don't ignore them, even if you have no risk factors or family history of cancer and have lived a healthy lifestyle.

People with existing conditions such as diabetes, cardiovascular diseases, chronic pulmonary diseases, psychiatric disorders, and dementia often have a different course of cancer detection and treatment, as well as more postoperative complications and a higher mortality. In some conditions, there is earlier detection because you are visiting your healthcare provider frequently. In others, especially psychiatric conditions, people may delay getting a diagnosis.

Various conditions may mean that healthcare providers are reluctant to do aggressive cancer treatment because your health is already fragile and you might not tolerate surgery, radiation, or chemotherapy. The cancer drugs might interact with the medications you are taking for your other condition. Your other condition might become worse, and this can make it difficult to complete cancer treatment.

For example, if you have lung disease, chemotherapy can result in lung inflammation and worsen your symptoms. Steroids and side effects of cancer treatment can affect blood glucose control in diabetes. In addition, with many conditions, you will have a slower recovery if you receive cancer treatment.

Cancer treatment is also difficult during pregnancy as the fetus would be affected by chemotherapy or radiation.

When to See a Healthcare Provider

There are very few symptoms that specifically mean cancer, so it's hard to know when you should be concerned. Any symptom that is new to you; that you have been living with, but is unexplained; and any change in bowel, bladder, or menstrual habits that is out of the ordinary for you is worth discussing with your healthcare provider.

Oftentimes, these symptoms turn out to be related to conditions other than cancer. But confirming that is essential to avoiding missing an early diagnosis.

Despite the importance of addressing cancer symptoms, many people delay talking to their healthcare providers. For example, a 2016 study found that the median time between noting symptoms of lung cancer and the eventual diagnosis was 12 months. People delay going to their healthcare providers for several reasons, including denial, fear of the diagnosis, or fear of being labeled a "complainer" or "hypochondriac."

If you note any symptoms, make sure to consciously admit the symptom to yourself and share your concern with a loved one you trust. Your healthcare provider wants you to bring up any unusual symptoms, and it can make a difference if cancer is found early.

The importance of early detection

Early detection is when cancer is found in its early stages. This can increase the effectiveness of treatment and lower the mortality rate.

Cancer screenings may help detect signs of cancer early. Some common cancer screenings may detect:

- Cervical cancer and prostate cancer. Some screenings, such as for cervical cancer and prostate cancer, may be done as part of routine exams.
- Lung cancer. Screenings for lung cancer may be performed regularly for those who have certain risk factors.
- Skin cancer. Skin cancer screenings may be performed by a dermatologist if you have skin concerns or are at risk of skin cancer.
- Colorectal cancer. The American Cancer Society (ACS) recommends regular screenings for colorectal cancer beginning at age 45. These screenings are typically performed during a colonoscopy. At-home testing kits may also be able to detect some

forms of colorectal cancer, according to a 2017 review of research.

- Breast cancer. Mammograms to test for breast cancer are recommended for women ages 45 and older, but you may choose to begin screenings at age 40. In people at a high risk, screenings may be recommended earlier.

If you have a family history of cancer or have a high risk of developing cancer, it is important to follow a doctor's screening recommendations.

While recognizing cancer warning signs may help people with cancer seek diagnosis and treatment, some cancers may be harder to detect early and may not show symptoms until the later stages.

Signs and symptoms of cancer can include:

- lumps or growths on the body
- unexplained weight loss
- fever
- tiredness and fatigue
- pain
- night sweats
- changes in digestion
- changes in skin
- cough

Specific types of cancers often have their own warning signs. If you are experiencing unexplainable symptoms, it is best to contact a doctor for a diagnosis.

How does cancer grow and spread?

Abnormal cell division

Normal cells in your body grow and divide. Each one has a life cycle determined by the type of cell. As cells become damaged or die off, new cells take their place.

Cancer disrupts this process and causes cells to grow abnormally. It's caused by changes or mutations in the cell's DNA.

The DNA in each cell has instructions that tell the cell what to do and how to grow and divide. Mutations occur frequently in DNA, but usually cells correct these mistakes. When a mistake is not corrected, a cell can become cancerous.

Mutations can cause cells that should be replaced to survive instead of die, and new cells to form when they're not needed. These extra cells can divide uncontrollably, causing tumors to form.

Creation of tumors

Tumors can cause health problems, depending on where they grow in the body.

Not all tumors are cancerous. Benign tumors are noncancerous and do not spread to nearby tissues.

But sometimes, tumors can grow large and cause problems when they press against neighboring organs and tissue. Malignant tumors are cancerous and can invade other parts of the body.

Metastasis

Some cancer cells can also spread through the bloodstream or lymphatic system to distant areas of the body. This is called metastasis.

Cancers that have metastasized are considered more advanced than those that have not. Metastatic cancers are often harder to treat and more fatal.

Treatment

Cancer treatment can include different options, depending on the type of cancer and how advanced it is.

- Localized treatment. Localized treatment usually involves using treatments like surgery or local radiation therapy at a specific area of the body or tumor.

- Systemic treatment. Systemic drug treatments, such as chemotherapy, targeted therapy, and immunotherapy, can affect the entire body.
- Palliative treatment. Palliative care involves relieving health symptoms associated with cancer, such as trouble breathing and pain.

Different cancer treatments are often used together to remove or destroy as many cancerous cells as possible.

The most common types of treatment are:

Surgery

Surgery removes as much of the cancer as possible. Surgery is often used in combination with some other therapy in order to make sure all of the cancer cells are gone.

Chemotherapy

Chemotherapy is a form of aggressive cancer treatment that uses medications that are toxic to cells to kill rapidly dividing cancer cells. It may be used to shrink the size of a tumor or the number of cells in your body and lower the likelihood of the cancer spreading.

Radiation therapy

Radiation therapy uses powerful, focused beams of radiation to kill cancer cells. Radiation therapy done inside of your body is called brachytherapy, while radiation therapy done outside of your body is called external beam radiation.

Stem cell (bone marrow) transplant

This treatment repairs diseased bone marrow with healthy stem cells. Stem cells are undifferentiated cells that can have a variety of functions. These transplants allow doctors to use higher doses of chemotherapy to treat the cancer. A stem cell transplant is commonly used to treat leukemia.

Immunotherapy (biological therapy)

Immunotherapy uses your body's own immune system to attack cancer cells. These therapies help your antibodies recognize the cancer, so they can use your body's natural defenses to destroy cancer cells.

Hormone therapy

Hormone therapy removes or blocks hormones that fuel certain cancers to stop cancer cells from growing. This therapy is a common treatment for cancers that may use hormones to grow and spread, such as certain types of breast cancer and prostate cancer.

Targeted drug therapy

Targeted drug therapy uses drugs to interfere with certain molecules that help cancer cells grow and survive. Genetic testing may reveal if you are eligible for this type of therapy. It may depend on the type of cancer you have and the genetic mutations and molecular characteristics of your tumor.

Clinical trials

Clinical trials investigate new ways to treat cancer. This may include testing the effectiveness of drugs that have already been approved by the Food and Drug Administration (FDA) but for other purposes. It can also include trying new drugs. Clinical trials can offer another option for people who may have not seen the level of success they wanted with conventional treatments. In some cases, this treatment may be provided for free. If you are interested in this kind of therapy, find clinical trials near you.

Alternative medicine

Alternative medicine may be used to complement another form of treatment. It may help decrease symptoms of cancer and side effects of cancer treatment, such as nausea, fatigue, and pain. Alternative medicine for cancer can include:

- acupuncture
- yoga
- massage
- meditation
- relaxation techniques
- Outlook

After you get a cancer diagnosis, your outlook can depend on a number of factors. These factors can include:

- type of cancer
- stage of cancer at diagnosis
- location of cancer
- age
- general health

Prevention

Knowing the factors that contribute to cancer can help you live a lifestyle that decreases your cancer risk.

Preventive measures to reduce your risk of developing cancer can include:

- avoiding tobacco and secondhand smoke
- limiting your intake of processed meats
- eating a diet that focuses mainly on plant-based foods, lean proteins, and healthy fats, such as the Mediterranean diet
- avoiding alcohol or drinking in moderation
- maintaining a moderate body weight and BMI
- doing regular moderate physical activity for 150 to 300 minutes per week
- staying protected from the sun by avoiding direct sun exposure and wearing a broad spectrum sunscreen, hat, and sunglasses
- avoiding tanning beds
- getting vaccinated against viral infections that can lead to cancer, such as hepatitis B and HPV

Meet with a doctor regularly so they can screen you for various types of cancer. This increases your chances of catching any possible cancers as early as possible.

Cancer and Diet

Cancer is one of the leading causes of death worldwide.

But studies suggest that simple lifestyle changes, such as following a healthy diet, could prevent 30–50% of all cancers.

Growing evidence points to certain dietary habits increasing or decreasing cancer risk.

What's more, nutrition is thought to play an important role in treating and coping with cancer.

Eating Too Much of Certain Foods May Increase Cancer Risk

It's difficult to prove that certain foods cause cancer.

However, observational studies have repeatedly indicated that high consumption of certain foods may increase the likelihood of developing cancer.

Sugar and Refined Carbs

Processed foods that are high in sugar and low in fiber and nutrients have been linked to a higher cancer risk.

In particular, researchers have found that a diet that causes blood glucose levels to spike is associated with an increased risk of several cancers, including stomach, breast and colorectal cancers.

One study in over 47,000 adults found that those who consumed a diet high in refined carbs were almost twice as likely to die from colon cancer than those who ate a diet low in refined carbs.

It's thought that higher levels of blood glucose and insulin are cancer risk factors. Insulin has been shown to stimulate cell division, supporting the growth and spread of cancer cells and making them more difficult to eliminate.

In addition, higher levels of insulin and blood glucose can contribute to inflammation in your body. In the long term, this can lead to the growth of abnormal cells and possibly contribute to cancer.

This may be why people with diabetes a condition characterized by high blood glucose and insulin levels have an increased risk of certain types of cancer.

For example, your risk of colorectal cancer is 22% higher if you have diabetes.

To protect against cancer, limit or avoid foods that boost insulin levels, such as foods high in sugar and refined carbs.

Processed Meat

The International Agency for Research on Cancer (IARC) deems processed meat a carcinogen something that causes cancer.

Processed meat refers to meat that has been treated to preserve flavor by undergoing salting, curing or smoking. It includes hot dogs, ham, bacon, chorizo, salami and some deli meats.

Observational studies have found an association between consuming processed meat and an increased cancer risk, particularly colorectal cancer.

A large review of studies found that people who ate large amounts of processed meat had a 20–50% increased risk of colorectal cancer, compared to those who ate very little or none of this type of food.

Another review of over 800 studies found that consuming just 50 grams of processed meat each day around four slices of bacon or one hot dog raised the risk of colorectal cancer by 18%.

Some observational studies have also linked red meat consumption to an increased cancer risk.

However, these studies often don't distinguish between processed meat and unprocessed red meat, which skews results.

Several reviews that combined results from multiple studies found that the evidence linking unprocessed red meat to cancer is weak and inconsistent.

Overcooked Food

Cooking certain foods at high temperatures, such as grilling, frying, sautéing, broiling and barbequing, can produce harmful compounds like heterocyclic amines (HA) and advanced glycation end-products (AGEs).

Excess buildup of these harmful compounds can contribute to inflammation and may play a role in the development of cancer and other diseases.

Certain foods, such as animal foods high in fat and protein, as well as highly processed foods, are most likely to produce these harmful compounds when subjected to high temperatures.
These include meat particularly red meat certain cheeses, fried eggs, butter, margarine, cream cheese, mayonnaise, oils and nuts.

To minimize cancer risk, avoid burning food and choose gentler cooking methods, especially when cooking meat, such as steaming, stewing or boiling. Marinating food can also help.

Dairy

Several observational studies have indicated that high dairy consumption may increase the risk of prostate cancer.

One study followed almost 4,000 men with prostate cancer. Results showed that high intakes of whole milk increased the risk of disease progression and death.

More research is needed to determine possible cause and effect.

Theories suggest that these findings are due to an increased intake of calcium, insulin-like growth factor 1 (IGF-1) or estrogen hormones from pregnant cows all of which have been weakly linked to prostate cancer.

Higher consumption of foods rich in sugar and refined carbs, as well as processed and overcooked meat, can increase your risk of cancer. In addition, higher dairy consumption has been linked to prostate cancer.

Being Overweight or Obese Is Linked to Increased Cancer Risk

Other than smoking and infection, being obese is the single biggest risk factor for cancer worldwide.

It increases your risk of 13 different types of cancer, including of the esophagus, colon, pancreas and kidney, as well as breast cancer after menopause.

In the US, it's estimated that weight problems account for 14% and 20% of all cancer deaths in men and women, respectively.

Obesity can increase cancer risk in three key ways:

- Excess body fat can contribute to insulin resistance. As a result, your cells are unable to take up glucose properly, which encourages them to divide faster.
- Obese people tend to have higher levels of inflammatory cytokines in their blood, which causes chronic inflammation and encourages cells to divide.
- Fat cells contribute to increased estrogen levels, which increases the risk of breast and ovarian cancer in postmenopausal women.
- The good news is that several studies have shown that weight loss among overweight and obese people is likely to reduce cancer risk.

Being overweight or obese is one of the biggest risk factors for several types of cancer. Achieving a healthy weight can help protect against cancer development.

Certain Foods Contain Cancer-Fighting Properties

There is no single superfood that can prevent cancer. Rather, a holistic dietary approach is likely to be most beneficial.

Scientists estimate that eating the optimal diet for cancer may reduce your risk by up to 70% and would likely help recovery from cancer as well.

They believe that certain foods can fight cancer by blocking the blood vessels that feed cancer in a process called anti-angiogenesis.

However, nutrition is complex, and how effective certain foods are at fighting cancer varies depending on how they're cultivated, processed, stored and cooked.

Some of the key anti-cancer food groups include:

Vegetables

Observational studies have linked a higher consumption of vegetables with a lower risk of cancer.
Many vegetables contain cancer-fighting antioxidants and phytochemicals.

For example, cruciferous vegetables, including broccoli, cauliflower and cabbage, contain sulforaphane, a substance that has been shown to reduce tumor size in mice by more than 50%.

Other vegetables, such as tomatoes and carrots, are linked to a decreased risk of prostate, stomach and lung cancer.

Fruit

Similar to vegetables, fruits contain antioxidants and other phytochemicals, which may help prevent cancer.

One review found that at least three servings of citrus fruits per week reduced stomach cancer risk by 28%.

Flaxseeds

Flaxseeds have been associated with protective effects against certain cancers and may even reduce the spread of cancer cells.

For example, one study found that men with prostate cancer taking 30 grams or about 4 1/4 tablespoons of ground flaxseed daily experienced slower cancer growth and spread than the control group.

Similar results were found in women with breast cancer.

Spices

Some test-tube and animal studies have found that cinnamon may have anti-cancer properties and prevent cancer cells from spreading.

Additionally, curcumin, which is present in turmeric, may help fight cancer. One 30-day study found that 4 grams of curcumin daily reduced potentially cancerous lesions in the colon by 40% in 44 people not receiving treatment.

Beans and Legumes

Beans and legumes are high in fiber, and some studies suggest that higher intake of this nutrient may protect against colorectal cancer.

One study in over 3,500 people found that those eating the most legumes had up to a 50% lower risk of certain types of cancers.

Nuts

Regularly eating nuts may be linked to a lower risk of certain types of cancer.

For example, one study in more than 19,000 people found that those who ate more nuts had a reduced risk of dying from cancer.

Olive Oil

Many studies show a link between olive oil and reduced cancer risk.

One large review of observational studies found that people who consumed the highest amount of olive oil had a 42% lower risk of cancer, compared to the control group.

Garlic

Garlic contains allicin, which has been shown to have cancer-fighting properties in test-tube studies.

Other studies have found an association between garlic intake and a lower risk of specific types of cancer, including stomach and prostate cancer.

Fish

There's evidence that eating fresh fish can help protect against cancer, possibly due to healthy fats that can reduce inflammation.

A large review of 41 studies found that regularly eating fish reduced the risk of colorectal cancer by 12%.

Dairy

The majority of evidence suggests that eating certain dairy products may reduce the risk of colorectal cancer.

The type and amount of dairy consumed are important.

For example, moderate consumption of high-quality dairy products, such as raw milk, fermented milk products and milk from grass-fed cows, may have a protective effect.

This is likely due to higher levels of beneficial fatty acids, conjugated linoleic acid and fat-soluble vitamins.

On the other hand, high consumption of mass-produced and processed dairy products are associated with an increased risk of certain diseases, including cancer.

The reasons behind these results aren't fully understood but may be due to hormones present in milk from pregnant cows or IGF-1.

Plant-Based Diets May Help Protect Against Cancer

Higher intake of plant-based foods has been associated with a reduced risk of cancer.

Studies have found that people who follow a vegetarian or vegan diet have a reduced risk of developing or dying from cancer.

In fact, a large review of 96 studies found that vegetarians and vegans may have an 8% and 15% lower risk of cancer, respectively.

However, these results are based on observational studies, making it difficult to identify possible reasons.

It's likely that vegans and vegetarians eat more vegetables, fruits, soy and whole grains, which may protect against cancer.

Moreover, they're less likely to consume foods that have been processed or overcooked two factors that have been linked to a higher cancer risk.

The Right Diet Can Have Beneficial Effects for People With Cancer

Malnutrition and muscle loss are common in people with cancer and have a negative impact on health and survival.

While no diet has been proven to cure cancer, proper nutrition is vital to complement traditional cancer treatments, aid in recovery, minimize unpleasant symptoms and improve quality of life.

Most people with cancer are urged to stick to a healthy, balanced diet that includes plenty of lean protein, healthy fats, fruits, vegetables and whole grains, as well as one that limits sugar, caffeine, salt, processed foods and alcohol.

A diet sufficient in high-quality protein and calories may help reduce muscle atrophy.

Good protein sources include lean meat, chicken, fish, eggs, beans, nuts, seeds and dairy products.

Side effects of cancer and its treatment can sometimes make it difficult to eat. These include nausea, sickness, taste changes, loss of appetite, trouble swallowing, diarrhea and constipation.

If you experience any of these symptoms, it's important to speak to a registered dietitian or other health professional who can recommend how to manage these symptoms and ensure optimal nutrition.

Additionally, those with cancer should avoid supplementing too heavily with vitamins, as they act as antioxidants and can interfere with chemotherapy when taken in large doses.

A Ketogenic Diet Shows Some Promise for Treating Cancer, but Evidence Is Weak

Animal studies and early research in humans suggest that a low-carb, high-fat ketogenic diet may help prevent and treat cancer.
High blood sugar and elevated insulin levels are risk factors for cancer development.

A ketogenic diet lowers blood sugar and insulin levels, potentially causing cancer cells to starve or grow at a slower rate.

In fact, research has shown that a ketogenic diet can reduce tumor growth and improve survival rates in both animal and test-tube studies.

Several pilot and case studies in people have also indicated some benefits of a ketogenic diet, including no serious adverse side effects and, in some cases, improved quality of life.

There seems to be a trend in improved cancer outcomes as well.

For example, one 14-day study in 27 people with cancer compared the effects of a glucose-based diet to those of a fat-based ketogenic diet.

Tumor growth increased by 32% in people on the glucose-based diet but decreased by 24% in those on the ketogenic diet. However, the evidence is not strong enough to prove correlation.

A recent review looking at the role of a ketogenic diet for managing brain tumors concluded that it could be effective in enhancing the effects of other treatments, such as chemotherapy and radiation.

Yet no clinical studies currently show definitive advantages of a ketogenic diet in people with cancer.

It's important to note that a ketogenic diet should never replace treatment advised by medical professionals.

If you decide to try a ketogenic diet alongside other treatment, be sure to speak to your doctor or a registered dietitian, as veering from strict dietary rules can lead to malnutrition and negatively influence health outcomes.

What exactly is the Dr. Sebi diet?

The plant-based diet is a form of alkaline diet, which was designed to purportedly help cells repair themselves through the combination of a restricted diet and supplements.

The designer is "Dr." Sebi, whose real name was Alfredo Darrington Bowman, was born in 1933 in Honduras. He was not a doctor, medical or otherwise, nor licensed healthcare practitioner of any kind (though his site calls him a "pathologist, herbalist, biochemist, and naturalist"). Entangled in a variety of civil and criminal litigation through his life, Alfredo was arrested for practicing medicine without a license. Bowman passed in August of 2016.

During his life, his diet had a number of celebrity fans, like Michael Jackson, but also was surrounded with controversy. He was known to deny that HIV causes AIDS and was in fact sued by New York state after claiming he had "cured AIDS" in 1993. He was told to stop making medical claims about his diet's benefits.

The diet prescribes a strict form of veganism and is based on the notion that all diseases have to do with a localized failure by the body's mucus membranes. Bowman proposed that by creating an alkaline environment, one can eliminate diseases.

As part of Bowman's diet, there's a"Nutritional Guide," which provides a list of foods you're allowed to eat (it's specific), along with some other guidelines.

His diet also advises taking Dr. Sebi "Cell Food" supplements. The program,for which there are gendered options, costs between $750 and $1,500.

Rules of the diet (per Bowman):

1. If the food isn't in his "Nutritional Guide," it is not recommended.

2. Drink one gallon of natural spring water per day.

3. Any Dr. Sebi products are to be taken an hour before "pharmaceuticals."

4. All Dr. Sebi products can be taken together without interaction.

5. Strict adherence to the "Nutritional Guide" (complete with supplemental products) gives the best results for "reversing disease."

6. No animal products, hybrid foods, canned fruits, seedless fruits, or alcohol may be consumed.

7. According to Sebi, using the microwave will "kill your food," so avoid using it.

What does it mean to alkalize the body?

An alkaline diet is based on the premise of controlling your body's pH with the foods you eat. Because the foods our body uses leave behind metabolic waste, the idea is that the waste can possess a pH varying from alkaline to acidic.

The human body has different pH levels in different areas to support specific physiological functions, with organs like the stomach being more acidic while blood is more alkaline. The homeostasis of pH in various organs and fluids is tightly regulated.

Through complex excretion and reabsorption mechanisms, our body has built-in acid-base balance via the lungs, kidneys, and buffer systems. One of the bodily products that is directly affected by the food and fluids we consume is urine. This is an example of a kidney-controlled mechanism for managing pH in the blood.

Do alkaline diets work?

The broader group of "alkaline diets" is based on the issue of metabolic waste, and the Dr. Sebi diet is one of many. The components of these diets are generally healthy enough in that they encourage eating more healthy plant-based foods, which would benefit most everyone. An alkaline diet typically criticizes or removes meats, seafood, eggs, dairy, sugar, processed foods, and wheat.

While these dietary changes would certainly yield health benefits for many (via sugar and calorie reduction, plus improved fiber intake and fruit and vegetable intake), the idea that diet patterns or components can materially influence our robust, built-in acid-base balance is unscientific.

There is no research behind alkalinizing the body, and science does not support the claims made by Bowman or similar alkaline regimens. Many studies on alkaline diets have been reviewed and meta-analyzed, and the results are in: Neither the alkaline diet nor its related "acid-ash hypothesis" have been shown to prevent or mitigate diseases. This lack of effect includes bone health and osteoporosis[1], cancer[2], and glucose and insulin responses

While it makes big claims, the diet is not proven. It may result in similar benefits to an alternate plant-based diet, for which the benefits are more well researched[4], but the strict diet plan does seem to lack protein sources.

When it comes to alkalinizing, Wendie Trubow, M.D., told mbg, "The claims, without research, should not be relied upon."

If you're thinking about trying a plant-based diet, there are plenty of benefits to look forward to. Here are some tips for starting your plant-based journey.

And if you're curious, here's the complete list of foods allowed on the Dr. Sebi diet:

- Vegetables
- Amaranth greens
- Avocado
- Bell Peppers
- Chayote (a Mexican squash)
- Cucumber
- Dandelion greens
- Garbanzo beans

- Izote (Cactus flowers/leaves)
- Kale
- Lettuce (but not iceberg)
- Mushrooms (but not shiitake)
- Nopales (Mexican cactus)
- Okra
- Olives
- Onions
- Sea vegetables
- Squash
- Tomatoes (only cherry or plum varieties)
- Tomatillos
- Turnip greens
- Zucchini
- Watercress
- Purslane (verdolaga)
- Wild arugula
- Fruits
- Apples

- Bananas
- Berries (but not cranberries)
- Elderberries
- Cantaloupe
- Cherries
- Currants
- Dates
- Figs
- Grapes (if seeded)
- Limes
- Mango
- Melons (if seeded)
- Orange (Seville or sour is best)
- Papayas
- Peaches
- Pears
- Plums
- Prickly pear (cactus fruit)
- Prunes

- Raisins (if seeded)
- Young coconuts
- Soursops (if you can find them)
- Tamarind
- Grains
- Amaranth
- Fonio
- Kamut
- Quinoa
- Rye
- Spelt
- Tef
- Wild rice
- Oils
- Olive oil (only uncooked)
- Coconut oil (only uncooked)
- Grapeseed oil
- Sesame oil
- Hempseed oil

- Avocado oil
- Nuts and seeds
- Hemp seeds
- Raw sesame seeds
- Raw tahini
- Walnuts
- Brazil nuts
- Seasonings
- Basil
- Bay leaf
- Cloves
- Dill
- Savory
- Sweet basil
- Tarragon
- Thyme
- Achiote
- Cayenne
- Onion powder

- Habanero
- Sage
- Pure sea salt
- Powdered seaweeds
- Pure agave syrup
- Date sugar
- Teas
- Burdock
- Chamomile
- Elderberry
- Fennel
- Ginger
- Raspberry
- Tila

Recipes

1. African Millet Salad

Ingredients:

1 cup adzuki beans, cooked and chilled

2 teaspoons mint

1 cup millet, cooked and chilled

1 cup red pepper, chopped

½ cup sweet onion, small diced

1 teaspoon celery salt

1 teaspoon tarragon

2 tablespoons toasted sesame oil

Directions:

In a large bowl, combine beans, mint, millet, red pepper, onion, celery salt, and tarragon. Mix well.

Drizzle sesame oil over salad.

Serve chilled.

2. Indian Arugula Salad

Ingredients:

3 cups cucumbers, peeled and chopped

2 cups plain nondairy yogurt

1½ cups tomatoes, chopped

1 cup fresh arugula, torn

1 tablespoon lemon juice

1 tablespoon flaxseed oil

1 teaspoon cardamom, ground

1 teaspoon apple cider vinegar

½ teaspoon sea salt

¼ cup toasted sesame seeds

2 teaspoons turmeric

¼ teaspoon cayenne pepper

Directions:

In a large bowl, combine cucumbers, nondairy yogurt, tomatoes, and arugula. Mix well.

In a small bowl, whisk together the remaining ingredients to create the dressing.

Toss the salad with the dressing.

Serve at room temperature.

3. Healthy Wild Atlantic Nori

Ingredients:

2 tablespoons toasted sesame oil

1 cup carrots, peeled and thinly sliced

½ cup daikon, peeled and diced

tablespoon tamari soy sauce

1 teaspoon lemon juice

1-ounce package laver (wild Atlantic nori) soaked in water for 1 to 2 minutes then drained and chopped fine

½ teaspoon fresh ginger, peeled and minced

1 scallion, chopped

Directions:

Add sesame oil to a skillet and sauté carrots over moderate heat for 5 to 7 minutes.

Add daikon, tamari, lemon juice, laver, ginger, and scallions. Cook an additional 1 to 2 minutes.

Serve at room temperature or chilled.

4. **Endive with Basil and Sprouts**

Ingredients:

1 cup curly or Belgian endive, chopped

1 cup Mesclun lettuce, torn

½ cup fresh basil, firmly packed

½ cup clover sprouts

1 cup fresh tomatoes, chopped

1 cup blueberries, as garnish

½ cup pears, diced, as garnish

½ cup toasted pumpkin seeds, as garnish

Directions:

In a large salad bowl, combine the endive, lettuce, basil, sprouts, and tomatoes.

Garnish with blueberries, pears, and pumpkin seeds.

Serve with a favorite salad dressing.

5. Cucumber-Arame Salad

Ingredients:

4 cups soaked arame

1 cup carrot, steamed and small diced

1 cup cucumber, sliced

½ cup yellow pepper, sliced

¼ sesame seeds

¼ cup apple cider vinegar

3 tablespoons extra virgin olive oil

3 tablespoons mustard

2 tablespoons date or maple sugar

1 tablespoon lemon juice

⅛ teaspoon cayenne pepper

Directions:

In a large bowl, combine arame, carrot, cucumber, pepper, and sesame seeds.

In a small bowl, whisk together the remaining ingredients.

Drizzle over salad and toss well.

Serve immediately.

6. Mango Salad

Ingredients:

10 ounces mango, peeled and cubed

4 ounces clover sprouts

1 cup walnuts

½ cup flaked unsweetened coconut

⅓ cup hazelnut oil

The juice of two lemons

1 teaspoon sea salt

Directions:

Combine all ingredients in a large mixing bowl and toss well.

7. Green Barley Split Salad

Ingredients:

6 ounces split peas, cooked

6 ounces spinach, chopped coarsely

6 ounces barley, cooked

6 ounces asparagus, cut into 1-inch pieces

3 tablespoons extra virgin olive oil

1 teaspoon minced garlic

½ teaspoon sea salt

Directions:

Preheat oven to 375°F.

Lightly grease a 4 x 8 baking pan with sunflower oil.

Combine all ingredients together. Toss and mix well.

Transfer to baking pan and bake for 15 minutes or until thoroughly heated.

8. Cheese-Apple Salad

Ingredients:

2 cups apples, cored and diced

8 ounces nondairy Swiss cheese, cut into strips

1 cup shredded nondairy cheddar cheese (4 ounces)

1 cup celery, blanched and diced

½ cup vegan mayonnaise

2 tablespoons lemon juice

⅛ teaspoon pepper

Lettuce

Directions:

In a large bowl combine the diced apples, cheeses, celery, vegan mayonnaise, lemon juice, and pepper.

Toss to combine and chill.

Serve on a bed of lettuce.

9. Arame Fennel Salad

Ingredients:

1 cup arame

½ cup fennel, chopped

½ cup daikon radish, shredded

¼ cup toasted sesame oil

6 tablespoons rice vinegar or apple cider vinegar

2 tablespoons lemon juice

1 teaspoon sea salt

¼ teaspoon freshly black pepper

2 tablespoons sesame seeds

Directions:

In a large sauce pan, cover arame with water and boil for 15 minutes.

Rinse under cool water.

Drain and measure 1 cup.

In a large bowl, combine arame, fennel, and daikon radish. Mix to combine.

In a small bowl, whisk together sesame oil, vinegar, lemon juice, salt, and pepper.

Pour over arame mixture, add sesame seeds, and toss well.

Chill for 1 hour before serving.

10. Fennel and Asparagus Salad

Ingredients:

¼ cup extra virgin olive oil

2 tablespoons fresh lemon juice

⅓ cup fresh orange juice

¼ teaspoon salt

¼ teaspoon freshly ground black pepper

⅓ pound endive, separated into leaves

½ pound asparagus, peeled into strips and blanched

1 pound fennel, white part thinly sliced

2 tablespoons fennel fronds, stemmed and chopped

2 tablespoons pine nuts, toasted

Directions:

Blend olive oil, lemon juice, orange juice, salt, and pepper until well incorporated. Set aside.

Combine endive, asparagus, fennel, fennel fronds, and pine nuts in a mixing bowl.

Drizzle dressing over salad and toss.

Serve immediately.

11. Mixed Sprout Salad

Ingredients:

2½ cups mixed crunchy sprouts

1½ cups sunflower sprouts

1 cup yellow pepper, sliced

½ cup heart of palm, quartered

½ cup artichoke hearts, quartered

2 beets, roasted and quartered

½ sweet onion, sliced

Salad dressing to taste

Directions:

In a large mixing bowl, add all ingredients except for salad dressing.

Drizzle salad dressing and toss.

Serve at room temperature.

12. Wakame Salad

Ingredients:

One package alaria (wild atlantic wakame), or 2 ounces

¾ pounds carrots, peeled and julienned

1 small red onion, chopped fine

3 tablespoons toasted sesame oil

2 teaspoons finely chopped peeled ginger

1 tablespoon black sesame seeds

The juice of two lemons

2 teaspoons tamari soy sauce

1 teaspoon sea salt

Directions:

In a medium sized saucepan, bring 1½ quarts water to a boil. Add the wakame and simmer for 20 minutes. Drain and chop fine.

In a medium sized saucepan, simmer the carrots in a couple of cups of water for 8 minutes, then drain.

Sauté the onion in the oil with the ginger for 10–15 minutes until the onions are translucent. Add the wakame, carrots, sesame seeds, lemon juice, tamari, and salt. Stir until well combined.

Serve over cooked white quinoa.

13. Spicy Arugula-Endive Salad

Ingredients:

1 cup beets, shredded

2 cups endive, chopped

1 cup baby arugula

1 cup yellow pepper, sliced

1 cup spicy sprouts

¾ cup fresh Italian parsley, chopped

⅔ cup red cabbage, shredded

¼ teaspoon cayenne pepper

1 cup fresh tomatoes, diced, as garnish

Directions:

In a large salad bowl, combine beets, endive, arugula, pepper, sprouts, parsley, cabbage, and cayenne. Toss thoroughly.

Garnish with diced tomatoes.

Serve with a strong lemon or vinaigrette dressing.

14. Watercress, Orange, and Endive Salad

Ingredients:

1 cup red, yellow, and orange bell peppers, sliced

1 cup endive, chopped

2 seedless oranges, sliced

1 cup sunflower sprouts

⅔ cup carrots, shredded

1 cup watercress

¾ cup fresh Italian parsley, chopped

1 cup fresh yellow tomatoes, chopped, as garnish

Directions:

In a large salad bowl, combine peppers, endive, oranges, sprouts, carrots, watercress, and parsley.

Garnish with chopped tomatoes, if desired.

Serve with a vinaigrette or light lemon dressing.

15. Asparagus Salad

Ingredients:

1 pound green asparagus

1 pound white asparagus

¼ cup extra virgin olive oil

¼ cup fresh lemon juice

¼ teaspoon sea salt

¼ teaspoon black pepper

¼ cup pickled ginger

1 teaspoon wasabi powder

Directions:

Trim bottoms of asparagus. Place in a medium pan and blanch 3 minutes.

In a small bowl, whisk together olive oil, lemon juice, salt, pepper, pickled ginger, and wasabi powder.

Arrange asparagus on a platter and drizzle with dressing.

16. Cucumber, Red Onion, and Dill Salad

Ingredients:

1 pound cucumbers, thinly sliced

1 medium red onion, thinly sliced

3 tablespoons fresh dill, chopped

¼ cup apple cider vinegar

2 tablespoons extra virgin olive oil

½ teaspoon garlic salt

⅛ teaspoon freshly ground black pepper

Directions:

Toss all ingredients together in a mixing bowl.

Serve immediately.

17. Garden Buckwheat Salad

Ingredients:

3 cups buckwheat noodles, cooked

1 cup broccoli florets, steamed 5 to 6 minutes

1 cup carrots sliced

¼ cup gomasio

2 tablespoons scallions, sliced

2 tablespoons golden raisins

2 tablespoons sunflower seeds

¼ cup toasted sesame oil

4 tablespoons tamari

Directions:

In a medium size bowl, combine noodles, broccoli, carrots, gomasio, scallions, raisins, and sunflower seeds.

Add sesame oil and tamari. Mix well.

Serve chilled.

18. Pear Beet Salad

Ingredients:

1 cup pears, sliced

1½ cups leeks, sliced and steamed 10 minutes

2 tablespoons fresh arugula, chopped

2 tablespoons fresh fennel, chopped

¼ cup olive oil

2 tablespoons prepared mustard

1 tablespoon fresh lemon juice

½ teaspoon cayenne pepper

½ cup beets, sliced and steamed for 15 minutes

Directions:

In a large salad bowl, combine the pears, leeks, arugula, and fennel.

In a separate bowl, whisk together olive oil, mustard, lemon juice, and cayenne pepper.

Toss beets in ¼ of the dressing and the remaining salad with the rest of dressing.

Arrange beets on plate and top with rest of salad.

Chill for 1 hour before serving.

19. Wild Rice Salad

Ingredients:

2 cups broccoli florets, blanched

3 cups wild rice, cooked

1 cup carrots, sliced and blanched

1 cup zucchini, diced

⅓ cup red onion, diced

¼ cup safflower oil

2 tablespoons fresh dill, chopped

¼ cup plus 1 tablespoon fresh lemon juice

1 teaspoon freshly ground black pepper

1 teaspoon sea salt

Directions:

Combine all ingredients in a mixing bowl and toss until well mixed.

Serve at room temperature.

20.Chickpea and Lima Bean Salad

Ingredients:

1 ounce dulse, dry

3 ounces green peas, cooked (chilled)

3 ounces chickpeas, cooked (chilled)

3 ounces lima beans, cooked (chilled)

2 tablespoons safflower oil

1 tablespoon dill, chopped

1 teaspoon tarragon, chopped

½ teaspoon sea salt

3 tablespoons lemon juice

Directions:

Soak dulse in hot water for 5 minutes, then rinse under cool water and squeeze excess water out.

Mix all ingredients together.

Serve chilled.

21. Mediterranean Cannellini Salad

Ingredients:

2 cups cannellini beans, cooked

2 cloves garlic, peeled and minced

1 tablespoon lemon juice

1 tablespoon thyme

1 tablespoon rosemary, chopped

2 scallions, chopped

6 ounces crunchy sprouts

⅛ cup balsamic vinegar or lemon juice

⅓ cup extra virgin olive oil to taste

½ tablespoon Dijon mustard

¼ teaspoon sea salt

¼ teaspoon freshly ground black pepper

2 cups field greens

Directions:

In a large bowl, combine beans, garlic, lemon juice, thyme, rosemary, scallions, and crunchy sprouts.

In a separate bowl, add the remaining ingredients, except for the field greens, and whisk to combine.

Drizzle over salad and toss.

Serve on a bed of field greens.

22. Indian Potato Salad

Ingredients:

2½ pounds assorted potatoes (a variety for color, taste, and texture)

⅓ cup crunchy sprouts

⅓ cup fresh parsley, chopped

½ cup olive oil

⅙ cup balsamic vinegar

⅛ cup tamari or wheat-free soy sauce

2 teaspoons cayenne pepper

1 teaspoon cumin

½ teaspoon sea salt

½ teaspoon freshly ground black pepper

Directions:

Bake potatoes at 400°F for 40 minutes, or until soft (insert fork to see how easily it goes through potatoes). Allow potatoes to cool completely.

Cut potatoes into large chunks, approximately 6 to 8 chunks per potato. Place potatoes in a large bowl. Add sprouts and parsley.

In a separate bowl, whisk together olive oil, vinegar, tamari, cayenne pepper, cumin, salt, and pepper.

Drizzle dressing over potato salad and toss to combine.

Serve chilled.

23. Curry Dressing

Ingredients:

12 ounces nondairy sour cream

3 tablespoons nondairy mayonnaise

4 teaspoons curry powder

1 teaspoon powdered ginger

½ teaspoon salt

Directions:

Put all the ingredients in a blender.
Process until smooth.

24. Salad Dressing with Garlic

Ingredients:

¼ cup apple cider vinegar

2 teaspoons dry mustard

1 teaspoon garlic, minced

1 teaspoon paprika

¼ teaspoon sea salt

¼ teaspoon freshly ground black pepper

1 cup safflower oil

Directions:

Put vinegar, mustard, garlic, paprika, salt, and pepper to taste, in a mixing bowl.

Add oil, beating with wire whisk.

Chill and serve over a favorite salad.

25. Creamy French Dressing

Ingredients:

2 cups extra virgin olive oil

1 clove garlic

2 teaspoons onion, grated

½ teaspoon dry mustard

⅛ teaspoon pepper

1 teaspoon paprika

1 teaspoon sea salt

¼ cup tomato juice

¾ cup vinegar

1 tablespoon egg replacer

Directions:

Place all ingredients in a blender and process until smooth.

Transfer to a tightly covered jar and store in the refrigerator.

26. Basic Vinaigrette

Ingredients:

¼ cup balsamic vinegar or lemon juice

1 cup extra virgin olive oil, to taste

1 tablespoon Dijon mustard

½ teaspoon sea salt

¼ teaspoon ground black pepper

Directions:

Whisk ingredients together.

Drizzle dressing over salad before tossing.

Serve immediately.

27. California Marinade

Ingredients:

3 ounces cauliflower florets, in bite size pieces

3 ounces bulgur, cooked (chilled)

3 ounces avocado, cut into ½-inch cubes

1½ ounces sunflower seeds

2 ounces shallots, chopped

1 ounce unsweetened shredded coconut

2 tablespoons extra virgin olive oil

1 teaspoon tarragon

½ teaspoon basil, chopped

1 teaspoon tamari

¼ teaspoon sea salt

2 teaspoons cider vinegar

Directions:

Steam cauliflower for 8 minutes.

Combine with the remaining ingredients and mix well.

Serve chilled.

28. Sautéed Kale with Shiitake Mushrooms

Ingredients:

¼ cup toasted sesame oil

1 pound kale, stems removed and cut into ribbons

1 tablespoon minced garlic

2 tablespoons minced ginger

1 large jalapeño, diced

⅓ pound shiitake mushrooms stems removed and sliced

1 tablespoon tamari

1 tablespoons agave

1 tablespoon sesame seeds

Directions:

In a skillet over medium heat sauté kale, garlic, ginger, and jalapeño in toasted sesame oil for 5 minutes.

Add mushrooms, tamari, agave, and sauté for 5 minutes.

Top with sesame seeds and serve.

29. Stuffed Avocado

Ingredients:

2 ripe medium avocados

½ cup chopped celery

¼ cup chopped fresh parsley

3 tablespoons lemon juice

¼ cup extra virgin olive oil

1 teaspoon maple syrup

¼ cup fresh basil

1 clove garlic, minced

Lettuce, carrot, and celery sticks for garnish

¼ teaspoon sea salt

Directions:

Remove the pits from the avocados and carefully scoop out the pulp, saving the skin. Vigorously whisk ingredients together with the avocado pulp in a large mixing bowl until smooth.

Fill the avocado skin with the mixture and chill.

Once chilled serve on a bed of lettuce with sliced carrot and celery sticks.

30. Apple Goji Walnut Millet

Ingredients:

1 cup millet

4½ cups water

½ cup unsweetened almond milk

½ cup chopped walnuts

½ cup chopped dried apple rings

¼ cup maple syrup

¼ cup goji berries

Directions:

Cook 1 cup millet in 4½ cups water in a medium-sized saucepan over moderate heat for 30 to 35 minutes.

Reduce heat to low and add almond milk, walnuts, apples, maple syrup, and goji berries. Cook for an additional 5 minutes.

31. Barley with Collard Greens and Leeks

Ingredients:

1½ cups barley

3 cups water

½ cup sliced leeks, white parts only

½ cup sliced mushrooms

½ cups sliced collard greens

1 cup chopped fresh tomatoes

¼ cup + 1 tablespoon extra virgin olive oil

½ cup sliced red bell peppers

¼ chopped fresh parsley

1 teaspoon garlic salt

½ teaspoon celery salt

½ teaspoons freshly ground black pepper

½ teaspoon dried oregano

Directions:

To cook barley, add 1½ cup barley to 3 cups of water. Cook covered for 20 minutes over moderate heat, until water is absorbed or until barley is done.

In a large saucepan, sauté the leeks, mushrooms, collard greens, and tomato in the oil over medium heat for 5 minutes.

Add the remaining ingredients, mix well, and sauté an additional 3 to 5 minutes.

Serve.

32. Coconut Nut Rice

Ingredients:

¾ cup brown rice

1½ cups water

½ cup unsweetened coconut, shredded

¼ cup raw cashews, chopped

1½ ounces dried apricots, diced

¼ cup raw sunflower seeds

¼ cup golden hunza raisins

1 cup coconut milk

¼ teaspoon cinnamon

1 teaspoon vanilla extract

Preparation:

Cook rice with 1½ cups water on high for 10 minutes, then lower heat to medium and continue cooking for 10 to 20 minutes until rice is done.

Combine brown rice with coconut, cashews, apricots, sunflower seeds, and raisins in a bowl.

Puree half the mixture in a food processor with coconut milk, vanilla extract, and cinnamon.

Add the rest of the rice.

33. Coleslaw with Fresh Fennel

Ingredients:

3 tablespoons lemon juice

2 tablespoons lime juice

4 cups green cabbage, shredded

2¼ cups fennel bulbs sliced very thinly

⅓ cup vegan mayonnaise

1 tablespoon picked relish

1 tablespoon fresh dill, chopped

1 teaspoon sea salt

¼ teaspoon black pepper

½ teaspoon apple cider vinegar

⅛ teaspoon cayenne pepper

Directions:

In a medium size mixing bowl, toss all ingredients.

Serve chilled as a salad or sandwich filling.

34. Mrs. Kartalyan's Rice Pilaf

Ingredients:

3 cups water

¾ teaspoon saffron threads

1 cup uncooked brown rice, short grain

3 tablespoons coconut oil

1 teaspoon fennel seeds

1 cup tiny rice pasta, in the shape of your choice, cooked

½ cup sliced almonds

Directions:

Bring 3 cups of water to a boil.

Add the saffron and reduce heat to simmer.

In a large saucepan, sauté the rice in the oil over medium heat until it turns light brown.

Add the saffron water and fennel seeds to the rice and cook on low heat for 25 minutes.

Stir in pasta and remove from heat.

Add almonds and mix.

Serve.

35. Brussels Sprouts with Tempeh Bacon and Toasted Hazelnuts

Ingredients:

2 green apples, peeled and diced

2 tablespoons fresh lemon juice

½ pound tempeh bacon (12 slices)

⅓ cup extra virgin olive oil

1 cup hazelnuts

2 pounds Brussels sprouts, trimmed and halved

¾ cup red onion, diced

1 tablespoon balsamic vinegar

½ teaspoon sea salt

¼ teaspoon black pepper

1 cup water

1 tablespoon pure maple syrup

Directions:

Preheat oven to 350°F. Roast hazelnuts until golden. Remove skins by rubbing them together. Set aside.

In a bowl, combine apples with lemon juice.

In a large deep skillet, sauté tempeh bacon in ¼ cup of extra virgin olive oil over medium heat, 5 minutes each side until browned. Remove from pan, chop finely, and set aside. Add Brussels sprouts, onions, balsamic vinegar, salt, and pepper to pan and cook for 5 minutes over moderate heat.

Add water and apples to pan. Cover and steam ingredients for 5 minutes.

Add tempeh bacon and continue to sauté for 10–15 minutes on low. Then add hazelnuts and maple syrup and serve.

36. Black Eyed Peas with Tempeh Bacon & Lemon Thyme Collard Greens

Ingredients:

8 cups black eyed peas

¼ cup extra virgin olive oil, plus 3 tablespoons

12 strips of tempeh bacon

3½ pounds fresh collard greens

11 cups Basic Vegetable Stock

1 cup finely diced yellow onion

½ teaspoon freshly ground black pepper

1 teaspoon sea salt

1 teaspoon lemon thyme

Directions:

Rinse black eyed peas under cool water, drain, and place in a large saucepan. Cover the peas and boil for 2 to 3 minutes. Remove the saucepan from heat source and cover. Allow the peas to stand for 60 minutes and rinse. Return to saucepan and set aside.

In a large skillet over medium heat, add ¼ cup of the olive oil. Add the tempeh bacon and flip while cooking 5 minutes each side. When golden brown, drain on a paper towel and dice very fine. Set aside.

Rinse collard greens thoroughly and remove the tough center stem from each leaf. Roll each leaf up and slice into 1-inch ribbons. In a large saucepan, add enough water to fill halfway and bring to a boil. Add the collard greens (they wilt quickly) and cook until tender, about 7 to 10 minutes. Remove the collard greens and place in an ice water bath and rinse. Return the collards to the saucepan and set aside.

Add 9 cups of the vegetable stock to the black eyed peas and cook for 10 minutes.

Add the chopped tempeh bacon and onions. Cook 25 to 30 minutes over medium high heat, covered. Cook until all water is absorbed and peas are tender. Set aside.

Add 2 cups of the vegetable stock to the collard greens and cook over medium heat for 7 to 10 minutes. Add the seasonings and stir to combine.

Serve the collard greens over the peas.

37. Kale and Red Potatoes

Ingredients:

1 tablespoon extra-virgin olive oil

1 leek, chopped

½ onion, peeled and chopped

1 clove elephant garlic or 3 regular cloves, chopped

2 cups kale, chopped

1 cup arugula, chopped

1 cup fresh watercress

¼ teaspoon powdered sage

2 russet potatoes, peeled and cubed

1 sweet potato, peeled and cubed

¼ cup potato water (see below)

Paprika as garnish

Directions:

In a saucepan, heat the oil over medium heat. Sauté the leek, onion, and garlic until soft, approximately 10 minutes.

Add kale, arugula, and watercress. Cook until tender, stirring frequently, about 5 minutes.

In salted water, boil potatoes until cooked through, 30 minutes.

Drain, reserving ¼ cup cooking water.

Place the potatoes in a medium size bowl, and add the sautéed greens, sage, and potato water and mash until moderately thick.

Garnish with a sprinkle of paprika.

Serve immediately.

38. Shiitake Basil Mashed Potatoes

Ingredients:

1 cup fresh basil, packed

½ cup extra virgin olive oil, plus 3 tablespoons

2 teaspoons fresh rosemary, chopped

Pinch of cayenne pepper

2 lbs Yukon Potatoes, quartered

¼ cup onion, diced in ½ inch pieces

1 teaspoon garlic, minced

½ pound shiitake mushrooms, stemmed and diced

1¼ teaspoon sea salt

¼ tsp white pepper

Directions:

Process basil, ½ cup olive oil, rosemary, and cayenne pepper in a blender and set aside.

Cover potatoes with water in a medium saucepan and bring to a boil for 20 minutes or until they are easily pierced by a fork.

Strain water from potatoes, place potatoes in a mixing bowl, and add the herb mixture.

Using a handheld mixer or masher, whip or mash the potato mixture.

In a skillet, add 3 tablespoons olive oil and sauté onion, garlic, shiitake mushrooms, sea salt, and pepper on low heat until lightly browned. Mash with potatoes.

39. Spicy Potato Bhaji

Ingredients:

⅔ cup extra virgin olive oil

1 large red onion, finely chopped

3¼ pounds Yukon Gold potatoes, sliced into matchsticks and reserved in water until ready to use

3 cloves garlic, peeled and chopped

1 tablespoon ginger, peeled and grated

1½ teaspoons turmeric

1½ teaspoons curry powder

1½ teaspoons cumin

1 teaspoon cayenne pepper

¼ teaspoon red pepper flakes

2¼ teaspoons sea salt

¼ teaspoon black pepper

1 x 10 oz package frozen peas

2 jalapeño peppers, seeds removed and diced

1 bunch scallions, sliced (about 1¾ cups)

1 cup cilantro, chopped

Directions:

Heat skillet for 3–4 minutes with oil over moderate to high heat. Add onions, potatoes, garlic, ginger, turmeric, curry powder, cumin, cayenne pepper, red pepper flakes, salt, and pepper. Sauté for 6–7 minutes. Cover and cook for an additional 2 minutes.

Add peas and cook for an additional 3–4 minutes, stirring constantly.

Add jalapeños, scallions, and cilantro and cook an additional 2–3 minutes.

40. Red Brazilian Rice

Ingredients:

1 cup chopped red onion

1 cup chopped fresh tomato

1½ teaspoons drained, crushed capers

¼ cup sliced large green olives

1 bay leaf

2 tablespoons extra virgin olive oil

1½ cups brown basmati rice

2 tablespoons pumpkin seeds

¼ teaspoon dried thyme

½ teaspoons freshly ground black pepper

1 teaspoon sea salt

Directions:

To cook rice, add 1½ cups rice and 4 cups water for 25 to 30 minutes over moderate heat, covered. Set aside.

In a large saucepan, sauté the onions, tomatoes, capers olives, and bay leaf in oil over medium heat until the onions are translucent, about 5 to 8 minutes.

Add the remaining ingredients and sauté another 3 to 4 minutes or until hot.

Serve with black beans.

41. Rio Rice

Ingredients:

2½ tablespoons toasted sesame oil

1 cup cauliflower florets, steamed

2 tablespoons fresh parsley, chopped

2 tablespoons toasted sesame seeds

⅓ cup black beans, cooked

⅓ cup brown rice, cooked

½ teaspoon tamari

½ teaspoon sea salt

½ avocado, sliced, diced, garnish

Directions:

Preheat the oven to 375°F.

Lightly grease a 4 x 8 inch baking pan with sesame oil.

Steam the cauliflower for about 5 minutes.

Combine cauliflower, parsley, sesame seeds, beans, rice, tamari, and sea salt. Mix well.

Transfer to baking pan and bake for 15 minutes.

Garnish with avocado slices, if desired.

Serve immediately.

42. Japanese Hijiki

Ingredients:

1 cup hijiki, soaked in water and drained

2 tablespoons toasted sesame oil

2 tablespoons finely chopped scallions

2 tablespoons diced red pepper

1 tablespoon tamari

Directions:

Sauté hijiki for 2 minutes over medium-high heat in sesame oil.

Add scallions, red pepper, and tamari to skillet and reduce heat to medium for 5 minutes.

Serve at room temperature.

43. Spicy Raw Thai Roll-Ups

Ingredients:

1 cup toasted coconut, shredded

1 cup cashews

½ lime or lemon, diced

3 teaspoons Thai chili paste

6 leaves young collard greens, trimmed and steamed

Directions:

In a food processor, mix together coconut, cashews, lime or lemon, and chili paste.

Drop 2 tablespoons of mixture on each leaf of greens and roll up.

Serve immediately.

Conclusion

There are many types of cancer in addition to those mentioned here. With an increased understanding of genetics, it's likely that the classification of cancers will improve significantly over the next decade.

The treatments for, and survival from, cancer have been improving in recent years, too. Ask your healthcare provider if you have questions about a specific cancer.

If you are diagnosed with a rare cancer, it may be worth asking for a second opinion at one of the large National Cancer Institute-designated cancer centers. These larger centers are more likely to have oncologists on staff who take a special interest in less common—but no less important—cancers.

If you have any of the cancer symptoms noted above or any symptoms not listed for that matter talk to your healthcare provider. At times it may be hard to determine the precise cause of a symptom. Be persistent. Symptoms are your body's way of telling you that something is wrong. If you aren't getting answers, ask for a referral or get a second opinion. Nobody knows your body or what is normal for you better than you do, and nobody else is as motivated to make sure it stays healthy.

Cancer is a group of serious diseases that are caused by genetic changes in your cells. Abnormal cancer cells may divide rapidly and form tumors.

Risk factors like smoking, drinking alcohol, a lack of physical activity, an unhealthy diet, having a high

BMI, and catching certain viruses and bacteria may contribute to developing cancer.

Screenings may help detect cancer early when it is easier to treat. The treatment plan and outlook for people with cancer can depend on the type of cancer, the stage at which it is diagnosed, and their age and general health.

Though there are no miracle superfoods that can prevent cancer, some evidence suggests that dietary habits can offer protection.

A diet high in whole foods like fruits, vegetables, whole grains, healthy fats and lean protein may prevent cancer.

Conversely, processed meats, refined carbs, salt and alcohol may increase your risk.

Though no diet has been proven to cure cancer, plant-based and keto diets may lower your risk or benefit treatment.

Generally, people with cancer are encouraged to follow a healthy, balanced diet to preserve quality of life and support optimal health outcomes.

medical concerns. open to 4pm

<u>416 946 2220 ext 2</u>

 after hours after 4pm
1-877-681-3057

carepath

Manufactured by Amazon.ca
Bolton, ON